The Invisible Makeup Technique

Your Guide for a "no-makeup" look

By

Marina Andreas

The Invisible Makeup Technique

Copyright © 2017

ISBN: 9781520990514

Warning and Disclaimer

Publisher Contact

Skinny Bottle Publishing

books@skinnybottle.com

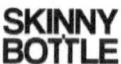

Your Guide for a "no-makeup" look

Make-up doesn't always have to be heavy and too bright to show beautiful or glamorous. In fact, the "no-makeup" makeup look has taken beauty enthusiasts by storm over the last few years and it still a very popular trend and why not? The "no-makeup" or natural looking makeup look has actually many benefits including:

- Enhancing your natural beauty

- Waking up and reviving your complexion with a natural finish

- Taking less time

- Wasting less amount of products and therefore saving money on the long-run

- Letting your skin pores breathe as you won't pile on thick layers of makeup that will stress your skin out and possibly clog pores.

If you have any skin issues, a light make-up application with good products won't do much damage to your skin, especially if you are using natural products and pigments.

The normal makeup look seems like a piece of cake but it's actually a bit tricky. as if you do a mistake with your application or choose the wrong products and colors, it will simply look unnatural.

If you've noticed many female (and male) celebrities in movies and magazines, their makeup looks naturally flawless and sometimes you even wonder if they are wearing make-up in the first place. If we exclude the screen and computer filters, their look shows that their make-up artist has done a great job at enhancing their features naturally. Professional makeup artists have actually mastered the technique and have been using it for years.

Now, you can use the same professional techniques, tools, and tricks, used by makeup artists all over the world for a light and natural look that will keep people wondering if you are wearing makeup or not. The most exciting part is that these techniques and tips will make you look good from all lights and angles—at daylight, nighttime, or even when taking a selfie or you are having a professional photoshoot. You can keep these a secret or share it your friends so they can look flawless and natural too.

Preparing the Skin

Preparing your skin for a natural makeup application is essential for getting a smooth complexion and a flawlessly natural makeup finish. Your face has to be as smooth as possible for the make-up to sit well on your skin, even though there is no need to go to any extremes to make it possible. However, you want to make sure that your skin doesn't turn bright red as this will defeat the purpose of preparing it.

Some quick fixes that will help smooth your skin's surface include:

Exfoliators. Exfoliators are probably the easiest way to get rid of dead skin build-up and smooth your skin's texture before you apply makeup. Still, you have to pay extra attention to the type of exfoliator you use to avoid any skin irritation or micro-bruising, especially if your skin is too sensitive. For best results, use a fine-granular exfoliator with sugar, fine salt, oatmeal, or any other fine granule scrub on damp skin. The scrub must be ideally creamy and leave no greasy film as this will interfere with the makeup application.

Enzyme Masks. Not all masks are suitable for preparing your skin for makeup application. In fact, since the majority of masks for the face are clay based, clay can sometimes make your skin look duller and drier than it actually is. For this reason, it's best to stay away from masks that are clay based, especially if you have a dry or combination skin type. One great alternative for smoothing and brightening your skin prior to a natural makeup application is using enzyme masks with fruit acids like AHAs and BHAs. Look for papaya and pineapple enzyme masks as these are suitable for all skin types and offer a natural radiant result. Apply these masks on cleansed skin and leave for at least 10 minutes or as long as it says on the package and then rinse off with water as usual.

Natural and artificial primers. Primers have been a very popular makeup trend over the last years and it's no wonder why. As their name suggests, they are used for priming and prepping the skin and making it smooth for a more even and flawless makeup application. Not all makeup primers though are created equal. Some are silicon-based while others contain more natural ingredients like for example corn starch or natural oils. If you want to get the best result possible, you need to choose a primer based on your skin type and your skin tone. For example:

• If you have a dull, dry, and mature skin with golden undertones, a silicon-based primer in lavender tone would be great.

• If you have rosacea, redness, and no visible wrinkles, look for a green-tinted primer which will help counteract the redness of your face without covering it all.

• If you have oily skin and your makeup tends to melt fast, look for a mattifying and oil-free primer in a transparent shade.

• Finally, if you have normal skin and no visible skin issues, you can go for an all-purpose primer in a clear shade.

Skin cleansing devices. Skin cleansing devices which rotate electronically or mechanically, are a great alternative to masks and exfoliators since you are going to use minimal to no product to cleanse your skin and remove sebum and dead skin cells. Clarisonic and Braun make great skin cleansing devices for this purpose. To make the most of these, turn them on and apply a cleanser on damp skin and use them at the same time till they foam for at least one minute prior to rising. The combo of the rotating brush and foaming cleanser will cleanse your skin deeply and more effectively than a simple cleanser.

Moisturizers and balancing creams. Moisturizers and day creams are sometimes necessary prior to make-up application as they help keep get rid of dry flakes and dull skin that will make the makeup look cakey and dry–which really isn't a pleasant and natural look. Like primers, though, you need to pay special attention to the formula and your skin type and avoid any heavy formulations that will just sit on top of your skin. It's best at this point to go for a lightweight moisturizer that offers the right amount of hydration without feeling heavy. Also, if you have oily or acne prone skin, you also need a moisturizer but it has to be oil free and balancing so it mattifies any oily spots, and moisturizes any dry flakes at the same time.

Blotting papers. Blotting papers can be used before and after makeup application to absorb excess oil, mattify the skin and make it look more poreless. If you have a problem with pores and oily skin, you'll have to blot your face regularly so you don't end up looking like an oil slick throughout the day. Keeping your oil at bay will also help prolong your makeup and make it last longer. If you don't have any commercial blotting papers available, a fabric softener tissue or tissue will work just as well.

Toners. Toners, apart from their tonifying skin properties can also get rid instantly of any excess sebum or moisturize and balance the skin out without leaving any residue. If you find that moisturizers or primers don't sit well on your face but you still want to prep your skin, toners are an excellent alternative. However, you also need to choose one according to your skin type as well. For example:

• If you have oily skin with no signs of dryness, look for a mattifying toner with witch hazel and a low alcohol concentration.

• If you have dry skin, look for a moisturizing toner with neroli hydrosol, rose water, or any other natural hydrating agent.

• If you have sensitive skin, avoid using any alcohol based toner and go for a pure herbal water like rose water or aloe vera juice which will hydrate and calm down any redness at the same time.

Essential Tools for Light and Natural Makeup Application

When it comes to getting the "no-makeup look" right, the tools are rules you are going to apply are very important for a flawless, effortless, and completely natural finish. Since you aren't going for anything heavy, you will not need much stuff but you need to pay attention to the few tools you'll use as well as how you will use them. If you have a wide variety of tools e.g. makeup brushes, isolate these first so you know first-hand which you are going to use to get that natural, "no-makeup" look

No 1: A foundation blender/sponge. Foundation blenders are much favored by the beauty community for offering a natural finish. Compared to foundation brushes or application with fingers, a foundation blending sponge can absorb excess product so it doesn't sit on top of your skin and blends more nicely with your natural skin's texture. Just make sure it is clear and sanitized before application so you don't transfer any nasty bacteria to your face, especially if you are suffering from any dermatological issues like acne or eczema. You may even use this damp, for an ever more natural finish.

No 2: A medium blush brush. If you've noticed already, most blushes with a mirror come with their own small brush for applying the blush to your cheeks. However, this brush is often too small and flat to give any natural effect. As a matter of fact, you may end up with unnatural and unblended stripes of blush instead of the natural flush you are going for. This is where you can use a medium round blush brush. Medium refers to a diameter that is close to 2-2.5 inches. Anything smaller or bigger than that will not give you a natural looking result. If you are going to use a powder blush, this brush is a mus t. The only exception is if you are using a liquid blush which already has a built-in brush for making small dots and then you can blend it with your fingers.

No 3: A base eyeshadow brush. Although makeup application has to be extra light on the eye area, you will still need a flat, medium size brush for applying any natural eyeshadow color for contouring your eyes. The brush should ideally have a size that covers the eyelid in 1-2 strokes so you can apply a base color in a nude-flesh tone. You can either use it dry, or wet for a smoother and more liquid-y finish.

No 4: A crease eyeshadow brush. A crease eyeshadow brush, as its name suggests, is used for applying an eyeshadow color to your crease, giving it more depth and shadow. Crease brushes are usually flat and very thin, or slightly large and round. This essentially depends on the size of your eyes and the look you are aiming for. Generally, the smaller the brush, the more precise the results—the bigger the more blended and wider. However, since there is also a blending brush that can blend things out, there is no need to worry if the crease line looks harsh on you.

No 5: Eye blender brush. Eye blender brush, as they call it, is used to blend the lines and creases of the eyeshadows so the result looks less harsh and more natural, without any obvious eyeshadow lines. The key here for getting the best results is to apply only a tiny amount of eyeshadow and then built-up if you see it needs more. Also, it's best to look for a fine brush with soft bristles (preferably non-synthetic) as it will be hard to work on the eyeshadow with a hard bristle brush and the result will look harsh and unblended.

No 6: Fine eyeliner brush. Eyeliner is not necessary when you are doing a totally natural, no-makeup look, however, fine lines of eyeliner from eyeshadow can do the trick of defining your eyes naturally without looking too obvious. This is the smallest and flattest eye brush for more precise and accurate results as eyeliners are the trickiest to apply. However, there are still some variations of it which give a slightly different result:

● Flat and wide eyeliner brush. This is one is a quite popular eyeliner brush which works with most eye shapes and is relatively easy to use. On the downside, it may not be useful for extra thin eyeliner lines.

● Angled eyeliner brush. This eye brush is flat yet slightly angled for a better coverage of the outer corner of the eyes and suitable for thin to medium lines.

- Fine tip eyeliner brush. This is the thinnest and smallest brush as it's literally a small tip made of a few fine hairs for drawing a very thin eye line. On the downside, this brush needs a steady hand as the line will get smudgy and uneven.

No 7: **Lip brush.** Lip brush can be used for applying any liquid or creamy lip product like lipstick, lip gloss, and lip cream. It's also necessary for protecting lip products from coming into direct contact with your skin and thus it's more hygienic, as long as you disinfect this regularly.

The brush has to be semi-soft, small and flat for the best and most precise results. Also, when using it you need to draw the outer edges first as if you are using a lip liner. Then fill in the rest of the product as it will be easier to fill in your lips to the perfect shape afterward.

Other optional brushes you can use are a concealer brush (for applying liquid or cream concealers) and a triangle makeup sponge for blending everything out and correcting mistakes

TIPS:

- Always use a natural bristle brush instead of synthetic for the smoothest and most natural-looking application. Additionally, natural hair makeup brushes do not get harder with time, as opposed to synthetic bristles which may come hard after time has passed.

- It is very important to wash or sanitize your brushes at least every couple of uses to get rid of nasty bacteria, oils, or makeup residue that may cause skin issues or even alter the final result. There are many makeup disinfecting sprays on the market that work in seconds, but if you don't want to invest in such products, washing your brushes regularly with a mild antibacterial soap and water is also a good alternative.

- When you use your brushes, unless time is an issue, you want to use light strokes with little product so you don't end up applying too much and then have no other option than to correct your mistake.

Top Makeup Techniques for Light and Natural Makeup Application

The following techniques for applying makeup for a natural and naked-looking result are not hard to follow but you need to pay attention for the most natural looking result. The steps are pretty simple as long as you know how to use each brush, Pay attention to the order of each step to get the best result. There are some basic steps that apply to all three techniques although there are also some small differences depending on the final finish you want to achieve e.g. radiant vs matte.

No 1: The Naturally Poreless Makeup Technique

This technique is for achieving a matte yet poreless and natural look that doesn't look cakey and fake. This makes a perfect choice for those with oil control issues and enlarged pores as it will help minimize their appearance without looking obvious. The basic steps for this technique are:

● Prep your skin using a mattifying primer. This will make your skin less shiny and help keep it nice and smooth before you apply your base. Apply only one drop to each section of your face and then begin to work all over your face, paying special attention to your creases and outer edges of your face that are hard to catch through initial strokes. If you have any skin blemishes, use a corrector individually on these spots (refer to the primer/corrector section in a previous chapter) to correct any skin tone issues that do not affect all your face. You can then dab a concealer or liquid foundation over these spots and then blend to match the rest of your face.

● Choose a light to medium coverage foundation with a soft matte finish. Notice that the finish has to be matte, but it should still be soft and easy to spread otherwise it will look cakey and unnatural. It's also wise to ditch heavy foundations as they will cake-up unless you are extra careful with your application. Ideally, you want to apply small dots of the foundation on key areas of your face like chin, cheeks, and forehead and then work these with your beauty blender. If you see any obvious foundation lines, gently blend with your fingers so they blend with your natural skin.

● Set your face with translucent powder. This will offer a more natural looking result than using a pigmented pressed powder. This step is also essential for blurring out your pores and making your makeup last more. Alternatively, you can use oil blotting paper to absorb oil and mattify the skin, if you still notice some shine but don't want to cake your face with powder.

● Use a powder blush in a natural rose shade (preferably not too bright, pink or dark mauve) with your blush brush. Make sure you use gentle strokes so you don't end up applying too much as this will make you look clownish. It's also better to build up the layers then apply heavy strokes from the first shot.

• Your eye makeup in this technique should be minimal or non-existent at all. However, if you want to add just a little definition to your eyes, use preferably matte eyeshadows in light nude colors like brown and beige on the eyelid, crease, and brow bone and blend well for a naturally smoky result.

No 2: The Ultimate Naked Face Technique.

This technique suits all skin types as it is something between matte and dewy and gives you that "your skin but better " look with a few subtle contouring touches. Among all other techniques, this is almost guaranteed to give you the most natural looking and undetectable results.

For this technique, you will need:

• A color correcting primer

• A BB or CC cream

• A translucent powder

• A 2 shade contouring set/palette

• A powder blush in a natural shade

• An eyelash curler

Here are the steps for this technique:

- Use a color correcting primer to instantly correct any skin issues prior to makeup application, as highlighted in the first chapter. You can use it either individually on spots that need the most correcting or all over your face, depending on the extent of the problem.

- Apply the BB or CC cream on top and blend with your foundation sponge. Make sure that the BB or CC cream you choose has light reflective or color adjusting particles so it looks more natural and less cakey or white. If your BB or CC cream has an SPF , you ideally want to go for a slightly darker shade as SPF will give your face an unnatural white cast, especially in photos with flash. This step is for evening out your skin tone and blurring imperfections while still letting your natural skin show through. Since BB and CC creams don't have any heavy coverage, you don't need any special technique to apply them and they are actually quite forgiving when it comes to mistakes.

- Use a cream contour palette with a contouring shade and a highlighter shade. To get the most natural looking result, your contouring shade has to be up to 3 shades darker than your natural skin tone while your highlight shade should be up to two tones lighter. Anything beyond this limit will most likely make your contouring efforts look unnatural. Also, the place of the contouring line is very important. Most contouring tutorials, if you search the web, call for using multiple contouring lines. However, to get the most natural looking and "naked" results, you will need to use the contouring shade in only 4 places: just beneath the apple of your cheeks, and on the sides of your temples towards your forehead and hairline. If you use any contouring to the lower parts of your face, you will exaggerate any hairs or strong jawline and your facial contours will look harsher. Keep the 4-contour line rule and you'll avoid that. Next, apply the highlight shade only an inch above your contour lines, with a more inward direction towards the inner part of your face. Use a foundation brush to blend the lines, preferably from inwards to outwards until they blend with the rest of your face and give you that natural sculpted look with no obvious lines.

• Use a powder blush in a nude brown or rose shade. Smile widely to locate the apple of your cheeks and apply the brush from the inside out with your blush brush, one gentle stroke at a time (2-3 strokes are fine for most cases). The placement of the blush should also be slightly above your previous contour and highlight lines for the best results and not underneath.

• Use an eye curler to curl your eyelashes and open up your eyes naturally without much mascara. For best results, heat the eyelash curler with a hair dryer for a few seconds and then curl your eyelashes from root to tip in an outward motion. Optionally, you can use a single coat of brown mascara for a natural definition to your eyelashes—just make sure that the mascara is not black or any other unnatural color and it's close to your own eyelash color for a natural and soft eye look.

• Finish off with a light layer of translucent powder or a makeup fixing spray to set your makeup and you are ready to go.

No 3: The Glowy-Natural Face Technique.

This technique is perfect for those looking for a naturally radiant and glowy healthy-looking skin that is not flat or matte. A great technique if you have a dull or dry skin tone and want to get a glimpse of that J-lo glow in a more natural way. The key to making this right and almost unnoticeable is to be light in your application of highlighting products and apply them at the right spots, as mentioned in the steps that follow.

For this technique, you will need:

- A light moisturizer or a color correcting primer (preferably of lavender tone)

- A foundation that offers a light coverage and a dewy finish

- A liquid highlighter with very fine micro glitters or oils

- A lip balm in a flesh or light red tone

- A foundation blending sponge.

Here is to get it:

- Prepare your skin with a lightweight moisturizer or a color correcting primer in a lavender or peachy tone. Apply specifically one small dot in each part of your face e.g. chin, cheeks, forehead and blend with clean fingers in circular motion.

- Grab the foundation. Like the previous step, make small dots for each part of your face and blend with a wet sponge. You can also blend with a foundation brush but a wet sponge will offer a more natural and blended finish with no obvious lines. If you still see any unblended parts, use your fingertips to blend everything out.

- Take your liquid highlighter and apply a very subtle line in your upper cheeks, temples, and inner nose. Blend with a sponge or with your fingers.

- Apply the lip balm to your lips for a natural looking and moisturized finish.

- Finish off with a setting spray/mist, sprayed approx. 6 inches away from your face.

Optional tip: This technique works best in places and occasions that aren't too hot or moist as such conditions may make your makeup melt in under a couple of hours. To preserve the dewy finish while extending the duration of the makeup, finish off with a very light layer of translucent powder after you apply all the main products. Results, of course, depend on the kind and brand of your primer as well as foundation as some seem to offer longer lasting results than others.

No 4: The Naturally Sculpted Face Technique.

This technique is based on a natural contouring process that makes you face look more defined and sculpted but in a way that looks almost invisible. It's basically a variation of a previous technique but with a few differences and a less shiny look. It is important to pay attention to all the products and shades you'll use as anything darker or lighter will simply look unnatural.

For this technique, you will need:

• A makeup primer that minimizes pores

• A light to medium coverage foundation with a natural semi-matte finish

• A contouring powder duo in a light highlighting shade and a contour shade that is just to two tones darker than your natural skin tone. Tip: the contouring shade must have cool or neutral brown undertones as anything too reddish or orange will look unnatural.

• A lip balm or non-glittery lip gloss in a nude shade.

Here is how to get it:

• Prime your face with the primer, making small dots and then blending with your fingers to distribute evenly.

• Apply the liquid foundation with clean fingertips and then blend with a makeup sponge.

• Begin the contouring process by using a medium eyeshadow or concealer brush (if you are using a cream contour palette) and make a 1-inch thick diagonal line, just below your cheekbones. Make also shorter lines on the tip of your chin and around your hairline and temples. Using the highlight shade highlight the upper cheek bones, inner bridge of your nose and inner forehead.

• Blend everything together and use a bit of concealer in outer areas that look too dark in contrast with the highlight shade. Finish with your lip balm and you are done!

Ideas for No-makeup Looks and Tips for Getting the Best Results

This chapter is all about getting specific "naked" looking results from looks and variations that cover 10 different skin tones–from the lightest to the darkest, with coloring product info and detailed steps on how to get the look shown in the photo. This chapter also features a natural seamless makeup look for each age group who wants to show off their natural beauty with little makeup.

No 1: Hint of Pink Look

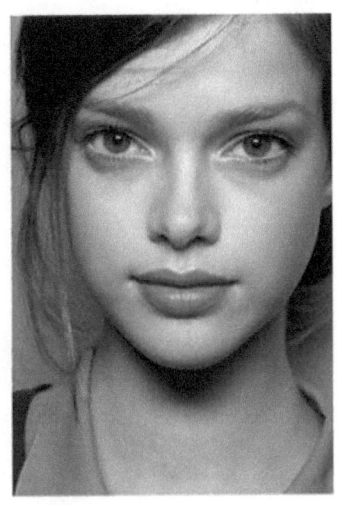

This is a great everyday look for extra light skin tones with cool white-pink undertones and a light eye color e.g green or blue. It has a subtle touch of cool-toned dusty pink which make extra light skin tones and eye colors like this look more interesting and fresh instead of ghastly pale or white.

To get this look, you will need:

• A BB cream with a natural semi-matte finish.

• A light reflecting concealer like Touch Eclat.

• A matte cool rose-toned blush like Milani's Tea Rose, Tarte's Dream, NYX blush in dusty rose, or Mac's Desert Rose

• A moisturizing chubby stick in a light mauve color like Clinique Chubby Stick in Roomiest Rose, Yves Rocher Mauve Tendre, and Maybelline's Baby Lips in Rose Addict.

- A brown volumising mascara like Max Factor's false lash effect in Dark brown and Inglot Color Pay Mascara in brown.

- A blush brush and a blending sponge

Steps:

- Moisturize your skin. Apply one to two layers of BB cream, making small dots and then blending with a sponge.

- Apply the light reflective concealer in darker skin areas like under eyes, upper lip, and temples.

- Take your blush brush and dip into the powder blush to absorb a light amount of product. If it looks too much, swipe a little on a tissue first prior applying to your face as it must look light and subtle. Smile to find the apples of your cheeks and apply the brush in an inward to outward motion.

- Apply a coat of brown mascara to the corners of your eyelashes

- Apply a layer of your chubby stick and rub your lips together to evenly distribute the product.

- Finish with a makeup setting spray.

No 2: Peachy-perfect natural make-up look

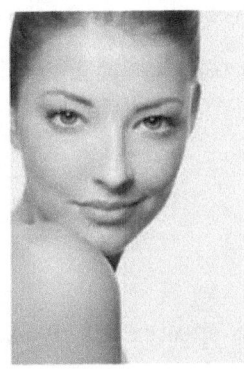

This look is perfect for light skin tones with cool peach or pink undertones and green, blue or gray eyes as it brings out these individual skin colors with very subtle and natural peachy hues. A great subtle daily look with a summery vibe.

For this look you will need:

• A tinted moisturizer like Nars Radiant Moisturiser, Laura Mercier Tinted Moisturiser, and Tarte BB moisturizer in light shade.

• A matte and sheer toned peachy-light coral toned blush like Mac's Gingerly and Clinique Cheek Pop in Peach Pop.

• A light reflecting concealer one shade lighter than your skin tone

• A dark brown mascara like Blinc Mascara in dark brown, and Max Factor Masterpiece in Black Brown.

• A peachy-orange chubby stick like Revlon's Rendezvous, the Style Hug Orange, or Clinique's oversized orange.

- A light matte navilla shade eyeshadow like Mac's Blanc type, Makeup Geek in Vanilla bean or NYX single eyeshadow in Skin.

- A medium warm brown eyeshadow in a satin finish like Mac's Texture, Anastasia Beverly Hills in shade Sienna, or NYX eutopia.

Steps:

- Apply the tinted moisturizer with a makeup sponge all over your face and neck.

- Use the light reflective concealer in your inner eye corner, in a triangle starting from your under eye area towards the cheek area, and in your inner nose and forehead. Blend with a sponge. Using medium flat eyebrows brush,

- Apply the peachy blush with a blush brush to your cheeks in a diagonal angle/line. Apply also a touch of the blush to the temples and outer forehead sides, in a horizontal V-shape.

- Apply the vanilla eyeshadow all over your eyelid and lower brow bone (it must not touch the eyebrow hairline). Apply the warm brown shade very lightly with a medium flat eyeshadow brush. Blend the two eyeshadows with an eye blender brush so that there are no harsh and obvious lines. Finish your eyes with a coat of dark brown mascara from root to tips.

- Apply a layer of chubby stick to your lips. Rub your lips together to distribute evenly.

Tips: for a slightly more brightening effect, you can use an extra light nude eye pencil on the inner rim of your eyes (white tends to look unnatural/obvious). This look doesn't require any heavy contouring so only use the blush and the highlighting concealer to add depth and dimension.

No 3: Snow White Wakes Up

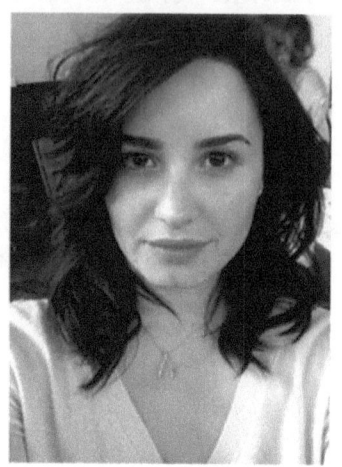

If you have dark hair and eye color but your skin is pale with neutral to warm undertones (like Katy Perry and Demi Lovato as in the picture), this seamless makeup look will ideally complement your natural colors while looking almost like you are not wearing makeup at all. It has a slight wash or red but it's so subtle that no-one would tell that you are wearing blush and lip balm. A great everyday look for winter and spring.

For this look you will need:

• A BB cream with a natural dewy finish and light coverage that lets your natural skin show through like Maybelline's Dream Fresh BB cream or Estee Lauder's DayWear BB cream.

• A light red cream/stick blush with a sheer non-glittery finish like NYX cream blush in red cheeks or Jordana Color Tint Blush Stick in shade 11.

• A light reddish pink lip balm like NYX juicy red, Nivea Strawberry, or Benefit Bene-balm.

- A clear mascara

- Eyebrow powder in a shade that's half a tone lighter than your natural hair color.

- Makeup setting spray.

- A flat foundation wedge sponge

Steps:

- Apply a thin layer of BB cream all over your face and neck. The BB cream must have color adjusting properties for the most natural looking result without looking too oily.

- Take a blush brush and deep into the cream blush or take a small amount of the product with clean fingers and apply directly to the apples of your cheeks. Make sure that the result looks rounder rather than horizontal and that there no obvious blush lines. This will also make your face shape look rounder if you have an oblong or square face.

- Apply the chapstick to your lips and rub them together.

- Apply one coat of clear mascara to your upper eyelashes for a bit of natural definition.

- If you have any sparse eyebrow spots, use an eyebrow powder and a small flat eyebrow brush to fill in the sparse spots. You can also tame any unruly hair with clear mascara.

- Finish your look with makeup spray/mist sprayed 6 inches away from your face.

No 4: Natural Asian Beauty

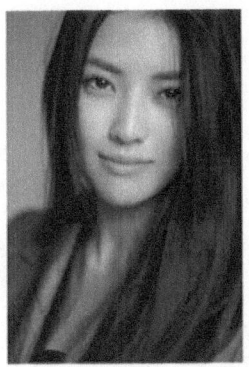

This natural looking makeup is perfect for those with light Asian skin and neutral undertones. It plays among the hues of peach and looks perfectly natural for any daily occasion–from office to going in out for lunch or shopping. It's also great for summer and spring due to its subtle brightening color combos.

For this look, you will need:

● A light reflecting BB cream with a natural and transparent finish

● A liquid or stick highlighter in a light pearly shade like Nars in Copacabana, RMS Beauty Luminizer (beauty editor favorite), and Revlon Skinlights in Pink Light.

● A liquid or cream blush in a light peach shade like Benefit's Cha Cha, MUFE cream blush in first kiss, or ELF Superstar

● A peach chapstick with a subtle wash of peach color like Maybelline's Baby lips in Peach Kiss, or NYX butter lip balm in Macaroon.

- Dark brown eyeliner like Revlon Colorstay in block brown, or Mac's technakohl in Photogravure

- Clear mascara

Steps:

- Optionally prepare your skin with a light moisturizer. If your BB cream already contains moisturizing properties, you may ditch this step.

- Apply the BB cream all over your face and neck, with your makeup sponge and blend any harsh lines with your fingers, if necessary.

- Apply the liquid/cream blush on the outer edge of your apples, towards the ears. The blush should be placed horizontally but towards the outer edge of your cheeks, not inwards (as shown in the photo).

- Apply the liquid highlighter on the line above your cheeks, your nose bridge, your temples, and your inner forehead. Blend.

- Apply a very thin line with your eyeliner as close to your natural lashes as possible and slightly extend it towards the outer corner of your eyes (approx. ⅓ of an inch outside the outer corner)

- Apply a coat of clear mascara to your eyelashes, from root to tip.

- Apply the peach lip balm to your lips directly and rub together to distribute.

Tips: You can use the same cream blush or tint to your lips too—the formula is not much different and you'll get almost the same effect.

No 5: A Touch of Spring Glow

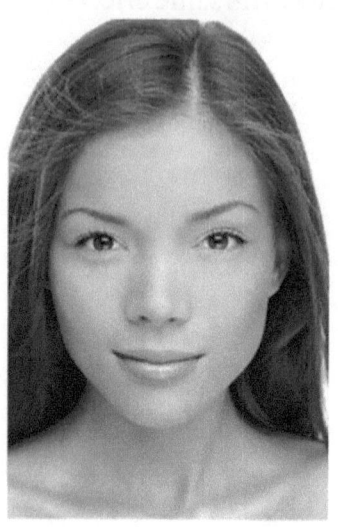

This look is a subtle representation of natural pink hues that remind the spring season. It is a perfect look for any skin tone and eye color, although it looks especially nice on light to medium skin tones with golden undertones and hazel//brown eyes, like the model in the picture. A nice look for any daytime occasion that doesn't look nor flat nor too dewy.

For this look, you will need:

• A CC cream with a natural semi-matte finish

• A matte powder blush in a peachy/honey shade like Jane Iredale Sheer Honey, Mac's Melba, or Loreal's True Match in Barely Blushing.

• A vanilla-colored satin eyeshadow, like Maybelline Chic Naturals in 15S linen, NYX single eyeshadow in cream cheese, or Colourpop eyeshadow in Girly.

- A light purple eyeshadow like Mac Purple Haze, Colorpop in Sneaking Suspicion, or Inglot in No. 392

- A translucent loose powder like Laura Mercier in Translucent Loose Setting Powder or Bobbi Brown, Retouching Powder.

- A nude peach tone lip tint like Revlon's Just Bitten, in Precious, Covergirl Oh sugar Lip Balm in Caramel, or Elf Lip Balm in Kissing Coral.

- An eyelash curler

- Clear Mascara

Steps:

- Apply small dots of the BB cream all over your face and neckline. Blend with the fingers or with a slightly dampened makeup sponge.

- Apply the blush with a blush powder in a gentle stroke, just over the apples of your cheeks.

- Apply the vanilla toned eyeshadow all over your eyelid and toward your brow bone. If it looks chalky, blend more or use a tissue to wipe any excess eyeshadow off.

- With your a medium flat eyeshadow brush, use the lavender eyeshadow from your middle eyelid to your outer crease. Blend well the eyeshadows with an eye blending brush.

- Use your eyelash curler from root to tips.

- Follow with a coat of clear mascara,

- Apply the lip balm on your lips and rub together.

- Finish off with a fine/light layer of translucent powder and a flat sponge.

No 6: Subtle Mauve Queen

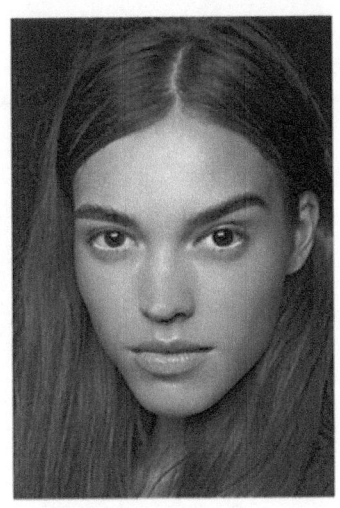

This subtle mauve look is great for those with naturally dark brown or medium brown hair and brown eyes and makes a great look to pull off in autumn, winter, and spring when you just don't want anything bright or fancy. The downside of this look is that it can accentuate tired looking eyes so make sure you use a concealer underneath to cover any puffiness and dark circles and use a cool-toned purple, like the ones suggested below so you don't end up looking like someone punches your eyes.

For this look, you will need:

- A color adjusting foundation with a natural semi-matte finish like Max Factor color adapt foundation, L'Oreal True Match, or Rimmel Match Perfection

- A light reflecting concealer like YSL touch Eclat, Diorskin Star concealer, or L'oreal's True Match, Touche Magique Concealer.

- A matte blush in a peachy-brown shade like Clinique's A-glow, Sleek Blush in Sahara, or L'oreal True Match blush in Nude Brown.

- A light plum/brown shade like NYX Cedarwood, Mac Sketch, or ELF single eyeshadow in Amethyst.

- A chapstick in cool-toned light mauve shade like Clinique's Fuller Fig, Revlon Colorburst Lip Butter in Candy (optional)

- A makeup setting spray

Steps:

- Apply small dots of the foundation all over your face and neck. Blend with a slightly damp makeup sponge or with your fingers.

- Apply the light reflecting concealer in a triangle under your eyes, and inner part of your nose and forehead. Blend well with your fingers.

- Apply the brush with a blush brush to the apples of your cheeks and towards your ears. Blush placement should start from the middle part of your cheeks (parallel to your iris) and towards your ears. For more depth and contouring, you can also apply a touch of blush to your temples, sides of the nose, and chin tip.

- Apply the mauve eyeshadow in your crease in light strokes, blending outwards towards your eye's outer corner–make sure though that it doesn't extend too much or the result will look unnatural.

- Apply the chapstick/lip crayon on your lips and rub together. If your skin has a natural mauve-y shade like the model above, you may ditch the step.

- Finish with makeup setting spray.

No 7: Natural Hawaiian Beauty

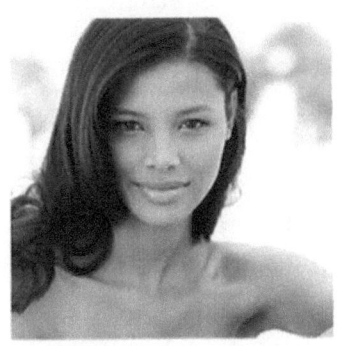

If you have medium/tan exotic skin and features (think Nicole Scherzinger), this natural look of subtle peach and sun-kissed honey hues will bring out your natural beauty. Other skin tones and eye colors can pull off this look just as well. A great look for spring and summer season.

For this look, you will need:

● A clear foundation primer with pore minimizing effects like Benefit Porefessional or Elf poreless primer

● A foundation with a natural traceless finish like Tom Ford Traceless Perfecting Foundation. Guerlain Tenue De Perfection, or Too Faced Born this Way.

● A cream.stick blush in a medium peachy shade like Jordana's Stick Blush Sun Kissed or Stila Convertible Color in Petunia.

● A lip gloss in a non-glittery transparent peachy hue like Maybelline's Baby Lips lip gloss in the coral craze, NYX lipgloss in Classic Coral, or Anastasia Beverly Hills in Melon.

- An eye kohl in a prune/mauve shade with brown undertones like Urban Decay, Glide On Eye Pencil in RockStar or Stila Smudge Stick Eyeliner in Tetra.

Steps:

- Prime your face with a primer by applying a few tiny (pea-size) spots on each part of your face and blend with your fingers.

- Apply 1-2 layers of foundation, again by making small dots and then blending with your face or fingers (provided they are clean).

- Apply a subtle layer of the cream blush or stick, directly over the apples of your cheeks making a circular rather than a stripe or horizontal shape. Blend well with a brush.

- Apply the eyeliner to your eyes and smudge lightly with a q-tip to make a light smokey effect, with no obvious lines. Tip: make sure that they eye pencil is placed on top of your lash line and not under your bottom lashes as that would make your eyes look red and tired.

- Finish your look with your lipgloss. For a more natural effect, lightly pat your lips with a tissue to absorb excess lipgloss. Your lips should look like they have a natural sheen/gloss but not too oily.

No 8: The Natural Sun-Kissed Goddess

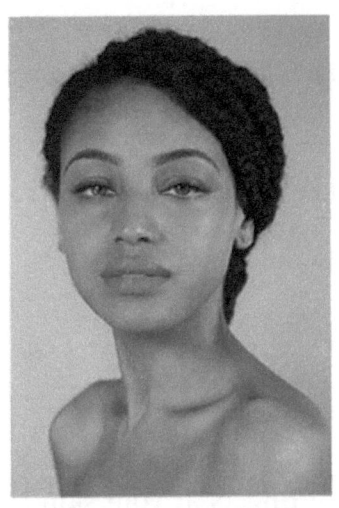

This look is perfect for tanned and dark skin tones with neutral undertones and hazel of brown eyes as it works with these colors harmoniously and gives a light sunkissed effect that is perfect for summer and autumn. A very subtle and natural look that doesn't look too matte or too dewy, for any daily occasion.

For this look, you will need:

•   A light coverage foundation in a natural/clean finish like L'oreal True Match foundation, Rimmel Clean Finish Foundation, or Body Shop Fresh Nude foundation.

•   A dark brown eye pencil/kohl like Urban Decay, Glide On Pencil in perversion, Mac Eye pencil in Coffee, or Revlon Colorstay Eye Pencil in black brown.

•   A light brown matte eyeshadow in neutral to warm undertones like Bobbi Brown eyeshadow in tan and Mac in Charcoal Brown.

- A nude brown lip liner like Milani Color Statement lipliner in Cocoa or Nyx lipliner in Nude beige.

- A nude brown lip balm/chubby stick like Clinique's in Heaping Hazelnut or Elf Essential Lip balm in nude

Tip: The lip liner shade has to be a tone darker than the lip balm to outline your lips with precision.

Steps:

- Apply the foundation making small dots, one in each part of your face and then blend with a sponge or clean fingers. If your skin is dry, make sure you apply a moisturizer or primer prior applying your foundation to prevent it from settling into fine lines.

- Apply the eye pencil just above your top lashes and smudge with a q-tip or eyeshadow brush outwards towards your crease, for a natural and very subtle smokey effect. Apply the medium brown eyeshadow just above your crease line and blend well with a circle small eyeshadow blending brush. They eyeshadow should almost reach your brow bone without actually touching the brows.

- Line your lips with the lip liner (make sure that is sharpened well for the thinnest and most precise lines). Apply the lip balm and rub lips together to distribute. If the lip liner looks too obvious or in contrast with lip balm hue, use a q-tip to blend or remove excess product.

Optional: This look doesn't require any blush or bronzer as a caramel skin tone like that can obviously stand on its own. You can, however, add a bit of dimension with a contour shade that is one shade darker than your skin tone and a highlight shade 1 tone lighter, making sure your blend well till there are no unnatural looking lines.

No 9: The Uber Natural Bronze Queen

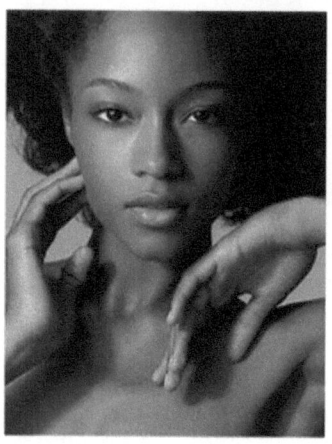

This look for naturally dark skin tones is so subtle and natural looking that it will make you look fresh and radiant without looking like you're wearing any makeup at all—almost like you have woken up liked this. Since your natural skin color is already dark enough, there is no need to put much color, especially for daily occasions.

For this look, you will need:

• A foundation primer like Smashbox Photo Finish Pore-Minimising primer or Maybelline Instant Pore Eraser Primer.

• A light to medium coverage moisturising foundation like Bobbi Brown Luminous Moisturising Foundation or Chanel Vitalumiere Aqua.

• A contouring kit with two shades: for contouring and one for highlighting, suited for those with dark skin e.g True Complexion Contour Palette medium to dark kit or Anastasia Beverly Hills Cream Contour Kit in Deep.

- A dark brown eye pencil like NYX in dark brown, Wet n Wild eye pencil in dark brown, or Urban Decay Glide on Eye Pencil in Demolition.

- A clear mascara

- A clear/no color moisturizing lip balm like Nivea or Maybelline Baby Lips. For a more natural alternative, you can use a bit of coconut oil instead.

Steps:

- Prime your skin with the foundation primer, paying special attention to dry areas like the sides of your nose and the area between your eyebrows.

- Apply your liquid foundation in small dots and blend with a makeup sponge.

- For the contouring technique: apply the highlight shade in light strokes over the inner parts of your face like your T-zone and temples. If you have dark under-eye circles, apply the highlight shade there as well in a triangle. Apply the darker contouring shade with a fine flat brush in the line just below your cheek bones (smile to see its natural contour) and blend all the lines together with a makeup sponge.

- Apply the eye pencil on the upper eyelid and smudge with a q-tip for a natural smokey effect (make sure that the effect appears like a natural crease or shadow rather than an obvious eyeliner line).

- Apply the lip balm or coconut oil to your lips for a touch of natural sheen.

No 10: The African Natural Beauty

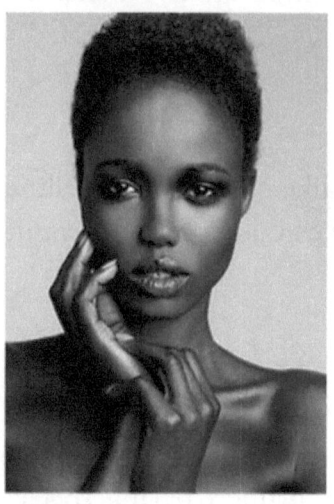

This look is perfect for the very dark afro skin as it brings out the natural beauty of this rare skin color without any obvious wash of color. A great polished look for all seasons and all daily occasions when you just want to look good with traceless makeup.

For this look, you will need:

• A light coverage foundation with a semi-dewy finish like Black Opal, True Color Foundation or Diorskin Star.

• A liquid highlighter in a nude-pearly shade like Benefit Moon Beam or NYX Liquid Illuminator.

• A cream blush in a medium tan shade with reddish undertones like Revlon Cream Blush in Nude or NYX cream blush in Tan.

• A soft black eye kohl like Chanel Ebene or Mac Eye Kohl Eye Liner in Smolder Black.

• A clear lipgloss or coconut oil

Steps:

• Apply the foundation in small dots over your face and neck and blend well with a dampened sponge.

• Apply the blush over your cheekbones in a diagonal direction. If you have an oblong face, place the blush in more circular shape.

• Make three small reverse triangles with your highlighter: two under your eyes (one under each), and one bigger reverse triangle on your forehead, to add light and dimension to your face. Blend well till everything looks nice and even.

• Take the eye kohl and apply from the inner corner of your upper eyelid towards the outer corner and the middle part of your under eyelash line, Smudge with a small circle eyeshadow brush or a q-tip for a mild smokey effect.

• Finish your look with a layer of clear lipgloss or coconut oil for a more natural shiny finish.

No 11: Teen and Fresh

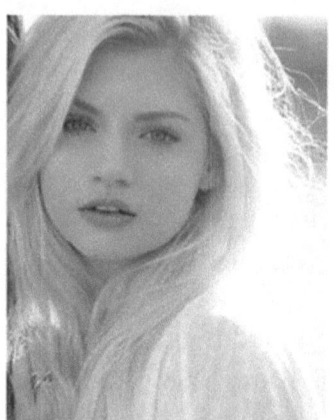

This look is designed to bring out the freshness and vitality of a young teen face with subtle rosy hues and minimal eye makeup as a teen's eyes are almost always sparkly and fresh on their own and don't need anything heavy. A perfect daytime looks for teens with light features and almost any skin tone except very dark skin tones.

For this look you will need:

•	A BB cream in a color adjusting tone like L'oreal Skin Beautifier BB cream anti-fatigue in Dr. Brandt Flexi-tone BB cream.

•	A transparent gel/liquid tint for cheeks and lips like Benefit's Posie tint or Soap and glory's checkmate lip/cheek tint.

•	A black brown mascara like Burberry's Effortless Mascara or Almay's Get Up and Grow in Black/Brown.

•	A light mauve.brown eyeshadow shade like Makeup Geek in shade Unexpected or NYX in beauty queen.

Steps:

•   Apply one layer of BB cream in small dots on all face parts and blend with a makeup sponge.

•   Apply the tint in small dots in your cheekbones and blend quickly with your fingers before it dries out and becomes hard to blend. Do the same thing with your lips, or use a lip brush for more precise results.

•   With a medium flat eyeshadow brush, apply the light mauve eyeshadow all over the upper eyelid and lightly towards the outer corner of the eyes.

•   Apply a coat of the black.brown mascara, paying special attention to the outer eyelashes.

No 12: The 20's Natural Diva

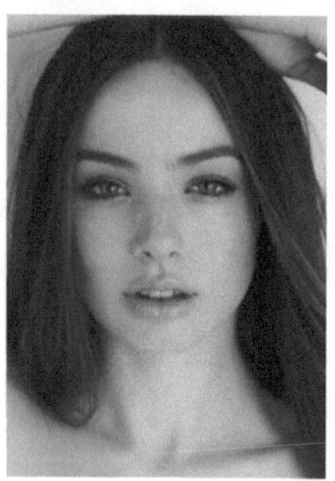

This natural light honey and sun-kissed look is perfect for girls in their twenties that don't have any heavy skin issues and want to achieve an almost traceless bronze-y look that is perfect for the spring or autumn season and suits a wide variety of skin tones, from lightest to darkest.

For this look, you will need:

• A light coverage foundation with a natural semi-matte finish like Too Faced Born this way or L'oreals True Match.

• A nude brown eyeshadow with warm undertones like Color Pop eyeshadow in Desert of Mac eyeshadow in soft brown.

• A grey-brown eye pencil like MUFE XL Aqua Pencil in Satiny Taupe or NYX Eyeshadow pencil in ash brown.

• A powder blush or a bronzer n a medium warm bronzey shade like Colorpop Bon Voyage or Channel Bronzer in Les Beiges 30.

• A lip balm in a nude pink transparent shade like Burts Bee's Honeysuckle or Elf Essential Lip Balm in Pink Princess.

Steps:

- Apply a thin layer of the liquid foundation making small stripes all over your face and neck and blend with a makeup sponge.

- Apply the matte blush with a soft blush brush from the parallel line of your eyes to the start of your ears.

- Apply the nude brown eyeshadow all over your upper eyelid and slightly above your crease. Get your eye pencil and line the upper eyelash line. Smudge with an eye blender blush to blend the line together with the eyeshadow.

- Apply a coat of the lip balm to your lips and rub together for an even looking result.

No 13: The Natural Busy Woman

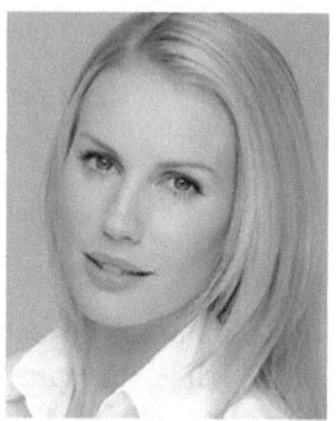

This complete natural and traceless makeup look will make you look polished and professional without having to wear much makeup as the colors are really nude and subtle–others will notice that you just look more fresh without being able to tell if you are wearing makeup or not. A perfect natural "no makeup" for a busy woman that doesn't want to show any signs of fatigue on her face.

For this look you will need:

•   A moisturizing BB cream or Tinted Moisturiser like Elf Tinted Moisturiser SPF 20 or Nivea 5 in one Beautifying BB cream.

•   A soft black lengthening mascara like Clinique's high impact or Shu Uemura Ultimate Natural Mascara.

•   A matte eyeshadow in a light peachy pink shade like Morphe Peekaboo or Mac in Shade girlie

•   A pink tone transparent lip balm like Nivea in shade watermelon or Revlon Just Bitten Lip Balm in honey.

Steps:

• Apply small dots of the BB cream all over your face and neck and blend with a makeup sponge.

• Use a flat eyeshadow brush and take a little eyeshadow (make sure that the brush doesn't pick up too much product) and apply to your upper eyelid, extending slightly towards your crease. If you have blue or green eyes, this will also add a touch of color and make them pop. Finish with a coat of mascara, paying special attention to your outer lashes.

• Apply the lip balm on your lips and rub together to distribute.

• Instead of using a blush, you can apply a bit of the lip balm to your cheeks for a more natural looking result.

No 14: Mature Natural Beauty

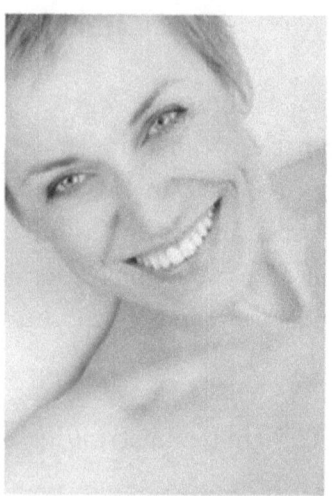

This nude makeup look is perfect for 45+ mature ladies who want to show off their natural beauty and not hide it under multiple layers of makeup. Instead of trying to cover up any fine lines or imperfections, this look will just blur them up so that they blend with the rest of your face. A great makeup look for any time of the day and spring or summer season.

For this look you will need:

• An anti-aging BB cream or tinted moisturizers like L'Oreal revitalift BB cream or Olay total effects CC cream.

• A matte powder blush in a peachy shade like L'oreal true match in Apricot Kiss or Laura Mercier Second Skin Cheek Color

• A soft black or brown mascara suited for daily wear like Bobbi Brown Everyday Mascara or Clinique High Impact mascara

• A sheer tone pink lip balm like NYX color lip balm in Merci or Burt's Bee's Tinted Lip Balm in rose.

Steps:

• Apply the BB cream or tinted moisturizer in light strokes in each part of your face (make a small line or dot) and blend with clean fingers. Let set and apply another layer.

• With a big blush brush, apply the blush to the apples of your cheeks. The blush should ideally be placed in a circular shape for a more youthful and fresh effect.

• Using the same blush, apply the color to your eyelids as well with a medium flat eyeshadow brush.

• Finish your eyes with a coat of mascara, focusing on your outer lashes.

• Apply the lip balm to your lips and smudge to distribute.

No 15: 60's Is The New Thirties

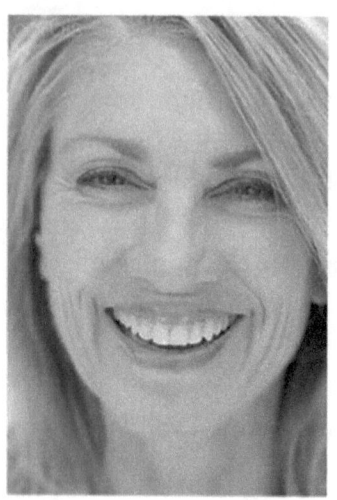

This look is perfect for highlighting the natural beauty of a 60+ face without trying to hide wrinkles in heavy layers of makeup as this may have the opposite effect. The hues used lean on the pink./mauve color spectrum and this is a perfect daytime spring and summer look for any skin tone and eye color.

For this look you will need:

•   A light to medium coverage wrinkle-blurring/anti-aging foundation like Maybelline Instant Age Rewind Foundation or La Prairie Anti-aging Foundation.

•   A light mauve matte eyeshadow like Lorac Mauve Eyeshadow or NYX in leather and lace

•   A dark gray eyeliner like Rimmer eye pencil in Stormy Grey or Urban Decay 24/7 glide on pencil in the mood.

•   A clear mascara

• A transparent dusty pink gloss (with no glitters) like Tom Ford lip gloss in Rose Crush. Or Maybelline in Mirrored Mauve.

Steps:

• Moisturize your face and apply one layer of foundation and blend with a slightly damp makeup sponge.

• Apply the eyeliner to your upper eye line from the middle part to the edges. Smudge lightly with a q-tip for a softer and more natural look.

• Apply a single coat of lipgloss to your lips and rub lips together to even out.

Natural Makeup Mistakes and How to Fix Them

Natural makeup may look very easy if you are a beginner, but it's actually challenging as the smallest mistakes in the technique or the products you choose can make your makeup look fake rather than traceless and natural. Here are the most common mistakes and how to fix them:

No 1: Your pores look huge with foundation

Enlarged pores are an issue that bothers women of all ages and especially those 30+ as aging gradually makes pores look more enlarged. If your foundation seems to highlight your pores and looks unnatural, this means that you either chose the wrong formula of foundation or didn't prime your face properly before applying your makeup. In the first case, look for a formula that claims it has pore minimizing or anti-aging effects that naturally blur imperfections and a lightweight coverage as heavier coverage foundations tend to exaggerate pores more. If your pores still look obvious, then it's time to pay attention to priming and preparing your face prior to applying your foundation. There are primers in the market that are targeted to minimize enlarged pores so apply a thin layer of the product before you proceed with the foundation.

Finally, a quick fix you can do is dabbing a bit of translucent powder or oil blotting paper on top of the foundation, especially if your skin pores look oily at the same time. Just make sure that you don't use too much powder otherwise you'll get the opposite effect.

No 2: Your foundation looks too cakey and dry

This the top mistake that women make which ruins a natural "no-makeup" look in an instant as nothing screams more "fake" skin than a cakey-looking foundation. One of the most common reasons why your foundation may look cakey is the wrong formula. In general, matte foundations tend to look cakier than other types of foundation finishes as they are frequently oil-free and don't have any sheen to them. Unless you have a problem with oily skin and acne, it is best next time to choose a foundation with a natural semi-matte or dewy finish.

Another common reason why your foundation may look cakey is the actual technique and application you use to apply it. If for example, you use a foundation brush and apply more than one or two layers without blending well, you might end up with a cakey looking result.

Finally, a cakey foundation can imply that your skin is dry or has dry patches and the foundation just sits on top and makes them look worse. The only choices here left is to either use a lightweight moisturizer, making sure it's properly absorbed by the skin or a moisturizing primer that will form an invisible layer to smooth out any rough patches and uneven skin texture.

Also, it's best to avoid using any powder on top of the foundation as it will make it look extra cakey–a little translucent powder is fine if you want to set your makeup but it's best to use a makeup fixing spray instead to avoid any cakiness.

No 3: Your foundation makes you look like a ghost

If your foundation makes you look like a ghost, then obviously you either chose a lighter shade than your skin tone or you have chosen a matte foundation with SPF. Matte and SPF foundation formulas usually contain ingredients and pigments like for example Titanium Dioxide that may give a gray or white cast to the skin, under certain lighting conditions. To avoid these, go for a formula that claims to reflect light or has color adjusting properties to match your skin tone. Of course, you need to check the color of the foundation first in both indoor and outdoor sunlight. Don't use your hands or neck to test it out as the skin there is usually lighter than the rest of your body and face. Instead, apply it directly to your face and if it seems to disappear without making you look whiter, then this is the right shade for you.

A quick fix in case your foundation is already white enough and you don't want to throw it away, is to use a bit of bronzer or brown eyeshadow. Take a few bronzer strokes with your fingers (or smash a bit your bronzer around the edges) and mix with a few drops of your foundation to achieve a darker shade. If you don't have a bronzer, a brown eyeshadow will have a very similar effect. If your bronzer or eyeshadow is loose, the application will obviously be easier as you won't need to shatter it to get a decent amount of powder to blend with the foundation.

Also, it's best to avoid wearing any kind of powder on top of the liquid foundation as it may add a ghostly white cast, especially when you take pics.

No 4: Your mascara or eyeliner smudges

When you suddenly realize that you have raccoon eyes, it's hard not to get panicked as it really looks funny and not in a good way. The no 1 reason why mascara or eyeliner smudges, even after minutes or a couple of hours, is because you used a non-waterproof or non-long-lasting formula. If you don't always have the time to fix things and avoid this from happening, it's best to go for a waterproof formula that will last for multiple hours without smudging. Go easy on the coats and avoid applying more coats of mascara. Too much product will smudge on your eyes faster. A foolproof option would be to wear clear mascara instead, especially if your eyelashes are naturally dark and you just want to give them a natural flare. Also, avoid applying mascara to your bottom lashes if they are naturally long or dense as the mascara will smudge your under eye area.

The same tips apply to keep your eyeliner from smudging. In general, going for waterproof or clear formulas and avoiding the application of products in the bottom lashes are the best ways to avoid smudging.

Now a quick fix to correct any smudging would be to dab a few dots of concealer around the area and clean up with a small makeup sponge of a q-tip. This works better than a makeup remover as a makeup remover will also remove product that you don't want to take off whereas this concealer tip will just fix the smudge in an instant without removing everything else.

No 5: Your eyelashes look too spidery/clumped up.

Spidey and clumped up looking lashes are another thing to avoid if you are going for a "no-makeup" makeup look. If your lashes look like a spider has crept in, then you have either used a high-fiber formula that adds fibers to the eyelashes in all sorts of directions or your mascara has the wrong type of wand/brush to coat them properly. A way to avoid this is to curl your lashes with an eyelash curler and then use a volumising mascara with a thick and feathered mascara wand/brush. The thicker the brush, the more naturally dense your eyelashes will look.

Also, make sure that you apply only up to two coats of mascara as any additional coat will clump lashes more.

Now in case you want to quickly fix this, unfortunately, you cannot do much. The only choices left are either to remove the mascara or use a clear eyelash wand to comb and separate them.

No 6: You have applied too much blush.

Applying too much blush is also another makeup mistake that will make you look clownish instead of natural and traceless. If you end up with two bright dots of blush on your cheeks, you have transferred too much product from the powder to the brush. Next time you use blush, make sure that you lightly dust it downwards to get rid of extra product and slowly build the blush in gentle strokes. It's better to go slow first than to regret it later.

Now, to quickly fix too much blush, the only way is to dab a bit of foundation or concealer around the edges of the blush and slightly blend it with your fingers till it has toned down. You ideally want to apply tiny dots and then blend instead of applying big swipes of concealer or foundation as they will wipe the blush off and you'll have to reapply it again.

Also, instead of a powder blush, you can also try using a cream or stick blush which is easier to control with fingers or a brush and blend. The only exception to using cream blushes is if you have very oily skin as this will make your cheeks look even oilier and brighter. It would also be wise to go on easy and apply small dots of the product first and then blend till you get a natural looking flush to your cheeks.

No 7: Your eyeliner and shadow look too bright or obvious.

If your eyeshadow and liner look too obvious and then it means that you haven't blended the lines enough.

Your eyeliner should look like a thick smoky and blended line in a natural earthy tone shade and not a fine straight line which makes it look too obvious. For this reason, it's best to go for eye kohls and pencils with a smudger than a liquid eye pencil and smudge with a brush or aq-tip any harsh and obvious lines, to give it a more natural shadowy effect. Blending well is the key for a natural eye makeup finish. It's best to avoid applying it over your entire eyelid and brow bone as this will make it look unnatural, especially if the color is dark. It's best to avoid any dark or unnatural colors and go for nude and earthy tones as this will offer the most natural looking results.

No 8: You face looks too oily or glittery.

On the opposite spectrum of cakey and dry looking makeup, is the makeup look that makes you look like a disco ball–which of course is unflattering unless you' are going to attend a disco party. This happens mainly for two reasons: the foundation is either too oily and dewy for your skin type, or you haven't properly primed your skin and set your makeup. In the first case, you can fix things by patting your face with oil absorbing.blotting paper and perhaps finish with a layer of translucent powder to set it and prevent it from getting too oily throughout the day. If your foundation looks glittery then you can't do anything because the tiny glitters will still show through even if you use powder on top. Therefore, next time check the ingredients and avoid anything that says it contains glitters and for a foundation that offers a clean semi-matte finish.

No 9: Your foundation has oxidized and looks orange.

Having a white ghostly looking face is one issue–but orange foundation that turns darker throughout the day is another problem. This situation is also called oxidization as the foundation pigments react to environmental factors like the sun and air and turn darker after a few hours. Some foundations, unfortunately, have an orange hue from the bottle, which might not be obvious in certain lights. Since the vast majority of foundations oxidize to some degree when exposed to outdoor conditions, one tip to prevent your foundation from oxidizing is to choose a shade that is half a shade lighter than your skin tone-careful though to not choose anything lighter than half a shade as you will end up looking white instead. A quick fix to prevent oxidization once you apply the foundation is to dab your skin with a very light layer of translucent powder. A concealer that is slightly lighter than your skin tone might also help brighten up instantly any dark skin areas.

No 10: Your contouring technique makes your face look dirty instead of naturally sculpted.

This may happen if you haven't blended the lines well or you chose a contouring shade that is too dark for your skin tone. As a general rule, it's best to go for a contouring shade that's up to two shades darker than your existing skin tone which has neutral brown undertones as orange and red based contouring shades will make you look unnatural under certain lights.

Additional Tips for a Totally Natural No-makeup Look

Apart from the previously mentioned basic techniques and looks in the previous chapters, there are some tips that will foolproof and improve your technique for a totally flawless and natural finish since in a "no makeup" makeup look, every little detail matters. Here they are:

No 1: Always check your makeup in different lighting conditions. It's easy to go overboard or ignore paying attention to the way you apply the makeup if your initial lights are blurry and "forgiving" of imperfections. Just because your makeup looks fine under your room lights, this doesn't mean it will look great and natural in other lighting conditions, e.g. sunlight or hospital light. Of course, it would be impractical or impossible to check your makeup in all different lights, but you should at least take a mirror and check your makeup outside to see if it still looks fine or looks harsh and unblended. If you are going to attend a night event it's best to also check your makeup under UV light.

You might also want to check how your makeup looks in photos under different lighting conditions. Try to make it a habit to take photos and look at them critically so that you can gradually fix any mistakes you are doing. The most common makeup issue that pops up in photos is a white cast on the skin (see the previous chapter).

Fortunately, you can find in the market some formulas that adjust to or reflect any type of light. These will most likely look great under any light as long as you blend everything properly.

No 2: Choose matte or creamy eyeshadows and blushes that don't contain any glitters.

Matte eyeshadows and blushes that don't contain any glitters offer a more natural finish for two reasons: first, they won't make you look like a disco ball and second, they won't settle on your fine lines and wrinkles as glitter-based products do. If you have mature skin it's best to avoid them entirely. Some products contain micro-glitters which are really subtle and give a natural looking sheen when used lightly, but too many layers of these can also look obvious, especially in natural sunlight.

If you don't want an entirely matte finish, which might also look unnatural, balance things out with a dewy or semi-matte foundation and a lip gloss or lip balm, like the looks I have shown in earlier chapters. Some formulas contain natural oils instead of glitters for a more natural finish so opt for these instead.

No 3: Use separate brushes for each part of your face (e.g eyes, cheeks, entire face) and avoid using the same brush for applying the same product.

You may think that you are saving time and money by using the same brush or same brushes to apply multiple products one after another, but what you are really doing is transferring bacteria and pigments from the last product to the next. You can't use the same brush, for example, to apply your foundation and then to apply cream blush as the brush will have soaked up liquid foundation pigments and they will clash with the pigments of the blush. Same goes with eyeshadow application unless you are using eyeshadows in complementary shades, like for example a light vanilla and darker beige. In this case, it is fine to use the lighter shade of eyeshadow first and then the darker one, with the same brush. However, the most natural looking and precise results are achieved by using a separate brush for each, as each eyeshadow brush is suited for a different part of the eye area.

Therefore, it's better to invest in buying the basic brushes as highlighted in chapter 1–many online retailers have incredible prices and discounts for these (some even sell the entire set for less than $10) so there is really no excuse to get a small 7 brush set to do all your makeup.

No 4: Groom and fill your eyebrows with a matte eyeshadow powder instead of a pencil.

Eyebrows should never be disregarded in a makeup look as they frame your face. If they are looking sparse on uneven, your face will look asymmetrical, sick, or aged. Many resort in using eyeshadow pencils to correct this, but these tend to draw too obvious and unnatural looking lines. If you are going to use an eyebrow pencil, one simple technique for getting a more natural looking result is to fill in any gaps and uneven spots by drawing small straight dots instead of long lines that begin from the start to the end of the eyebrow and then blending these with an eyebrow brush (also called a spoolie). The eyebrow brush should be used lightly from inwards to outwards for the best result. Many pencils come with their own small brush on the other side of the pencil so you don't need to buy a separate one unless it's too small and doesn't fit the size of your eyebrows.

If you are using an eyeshadow powder, which tends to offer a more-natural-looking finish, do the same technique with the dots and blend with an eyebrow brush/wand.

The shade you choose also plays a big part on how natural your eyebrows will look. In general, it's best to go for a half shade lighter if your eyebrows are dark brown or black and a shade darker in you have blonde eyebrows e.g. light brown instead of golden blonde. If you blend the lines properly, your natural eyebrow color and border will look clear and defined without looking that you used an eyebrow pencil or eyeshadow. If there are any stray hairs popping outside the border than ruin the shape of your eyebrows, pluck them or shave them with an eyebrow shaver for a more polished finish.

You Are a Song

Getting that no-makeup look may sound like an easy task to those who haven't tried it yet. Once you are at it, you will likely going to realize that it is much harder than you thought it would be.

If your face was a song, the no-makeup long would be just a vocal and a piano. The opposite of that, the makeup look, would be a vocal, backing vocals, pianos, guitars, drums and synths. The presence of many instruments creates a wall of sound where small mistakes in performances can hide. However, if there is only a vocal and a piano, these mistakes can no longer hide.

Just like a song, it is harder to create a polished look when you have to be subtle and use limited makeup quantities. The no-makeup look is much less forgiving on mistakes, so you need to know what you are doing or be willing to experiment and learn.

If you should remember one thing from reading this book, remember this. In all occasions and looks, the most common tip to achieve a traceless finish is to blend very well till there are no harsh lines and only use light layers of products that offer a sheer wash of color and not heavy coverage.

Win a free

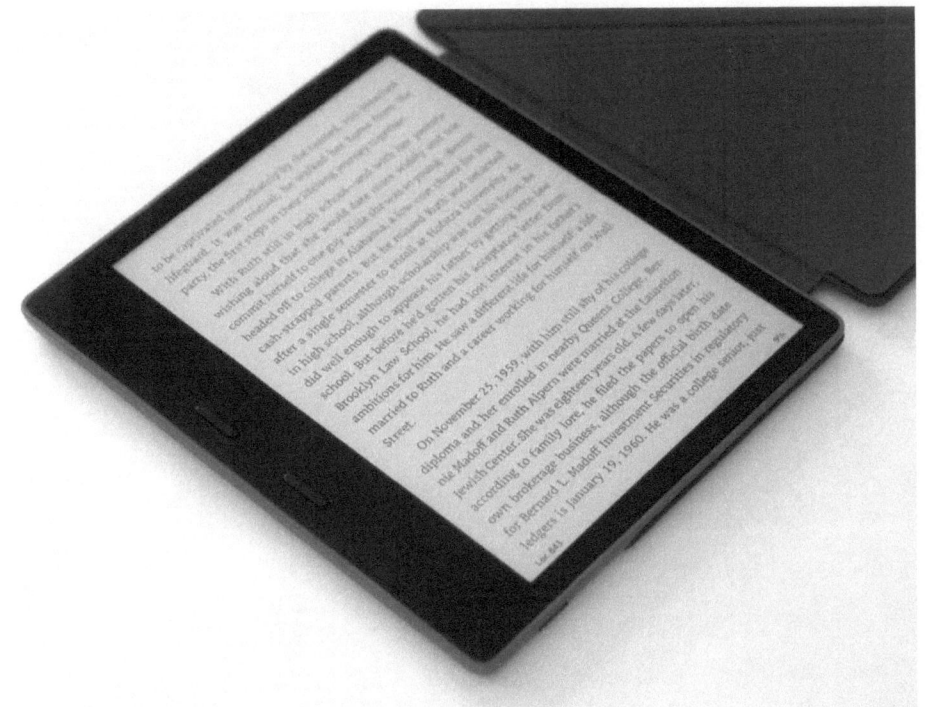

kindle
OASIS

Let us know what you thought of this book to enter the sweepstake at:

http://booksfor.review/invisiblemakeup